The Super Simple Mediterranean Cooking Guide

Irresistible Meals To Improve Your Health and Boost Your Metabolism

Alison Russell

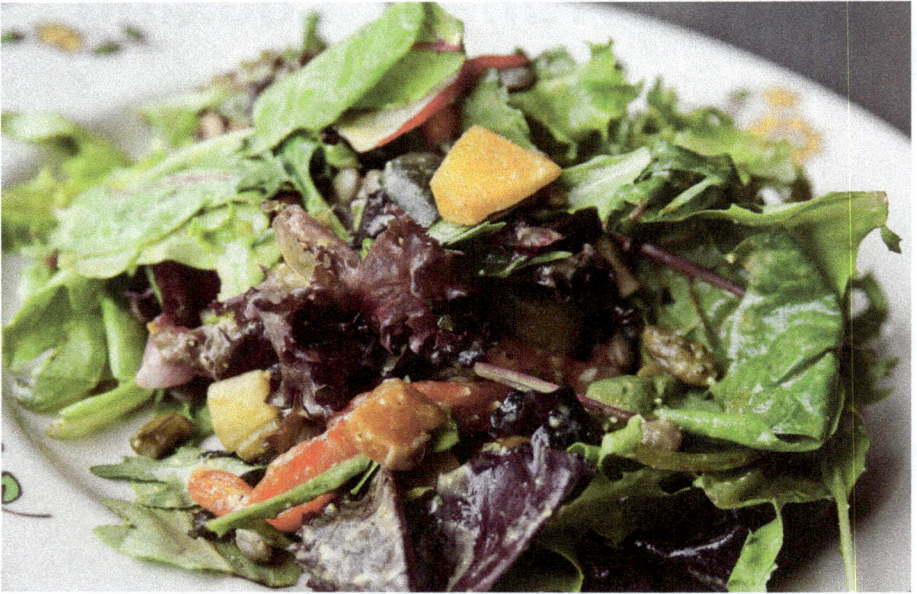

advice. The content within this book has been derived from various sources. Please consult a licensed professional before attempting any techniques outlined in this book.

By reading this document, the reader agrees that under no circumstances is the author responsible for any losses, direct or indirect, which are incurred as a result of the use of information contained within this document, including, but not limited to, — errors, omissions, or inaccuracies.

Table of contents

Breakfasts

Creamy Breakfast Bulgur with Berries

Prep time: 2 minutes | Cook time: 10 minutes | Serves 2

½ cup medium-grain bulgur wheat

1 cup water

Pinch sea salt

¼ cup unsweetened almond milk

1 teaspoon pure vanilla extract

¼ teaspoon ground cinnamon

1 cup fresh berries of your choice

1. Put the bulgur in a medium saucepan with the water and sea salt, and bring to a boil.
2. Cover, remove from heat, and let stand for 10 minutes until water is absorbed.
3. Stir in the milk, vanilla, and cinnamon until fully incorporated. Divide between 2 bowls and top with the fresh berries to serve.

Per Serving

calories: 173 | fat: 1.6g | protein: 5.7g | carbs: 34.0g | fiber: 6.0g | sodium: 197mg

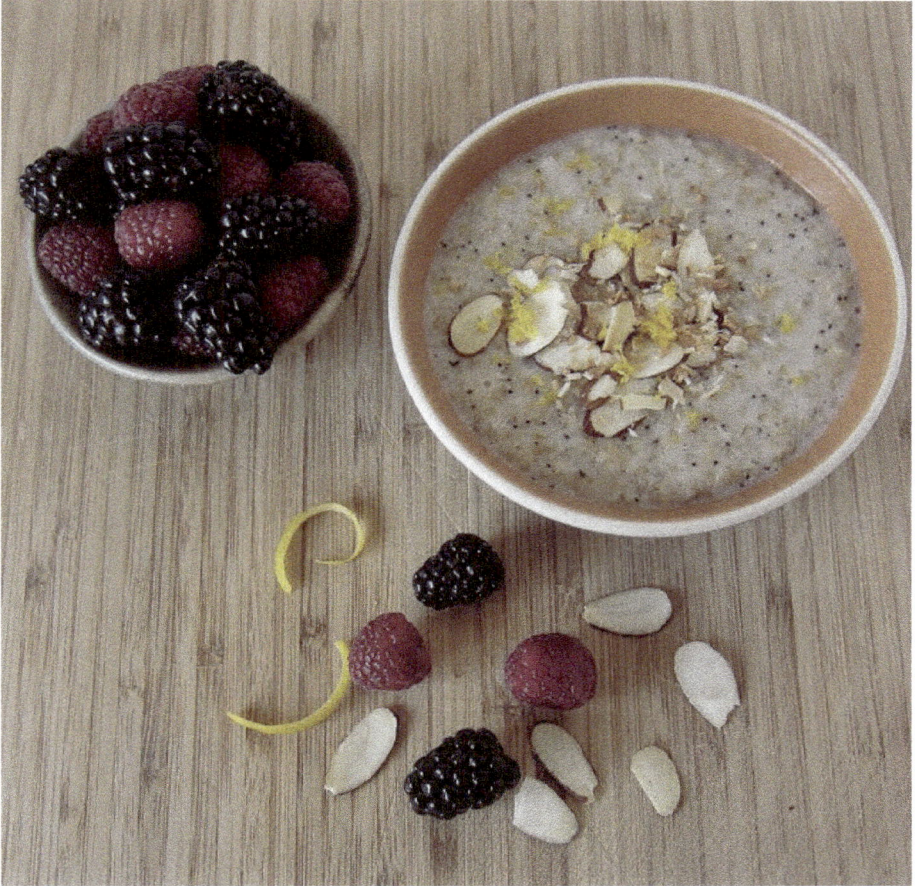

Basil Scrambled Eggs

Prep time: 5 minutes | Cook time: 8 minutes | Serves 2

4 large eggs

2 tablespoons grated Gruyère cheese

2 tablespoons finely chopped fresh basil

1 tablespoon plain Greek yogurt

1 tablespoon olive oil

2 cloves garlic, minced

Sea salt and freshly ground pepper, to taste

1. In a large bowl, beat together the eggs, cheese, basil, and yogurt with a whisk until just combined.
2. Heat the oil in a large, heavy nonstick skillet over medium-low heat. Add the garlic and cook until golden, about 1 minute.
3. Pour the egg mixture into the skillet over the garlic. Work the eggs continuously and cook until fluffy and soft.
4. Season with sea salt and freshly ground pepper to taste. Divide between 2 plates and serve immediately.

Per Serving

calories: 243 | fat: 19.7g | protein: 15.6g | carbs: 3.4g | fiber: 0.1g | sodium: 568mg

Kale and Apple Smoothie

Prep time: 5 minutes | Cook time: 0 minutes | Serves 2

2 cups shredded kale

1 cup unsweetened almond milk

¼ cup 2 percent plain Greek yogurt

½ Granny Smith apple, unpeeled, cored and chopped

½ avocado, diced 3 ice cubes

1. Put all ingredients in a blender and blend until smooth and thick.
2. Pour into two glasses and serve immediately.

Per Serving

calories: 177 | fat: 6.8g | protein: 8.2g | carbs: 22.0g | fiber: 4.1g | sodium: 112mg

Cinnamon Oatmeal with Dried Cranberries

Prep time: 5 minutes | Cook time: 8 minutes | Serves 2

1 cup almond milk   1 cup old-fashioned oats

1 cup water   ½ cup dried cranberries

Pinch sea salt   1 teaspoon ground cinnamon

1. In a medium saucepan over high heat, bring the almond milk, water, and salt to a boil.
2. Stir in the oats, cranberries, and cinnamon. Reduce the heat to medium and cook for 5 minutes, stirring occasionally.
3. Remove the oatmeal from the heat. Cover and let it stand for 3 minutes.
4. Stir before serving.

Per Serving

calories: 107 | fat: 2.1g | protein: 3.2g | carbs: 18.2g | fiber: 4.1g | sodium: 122mg

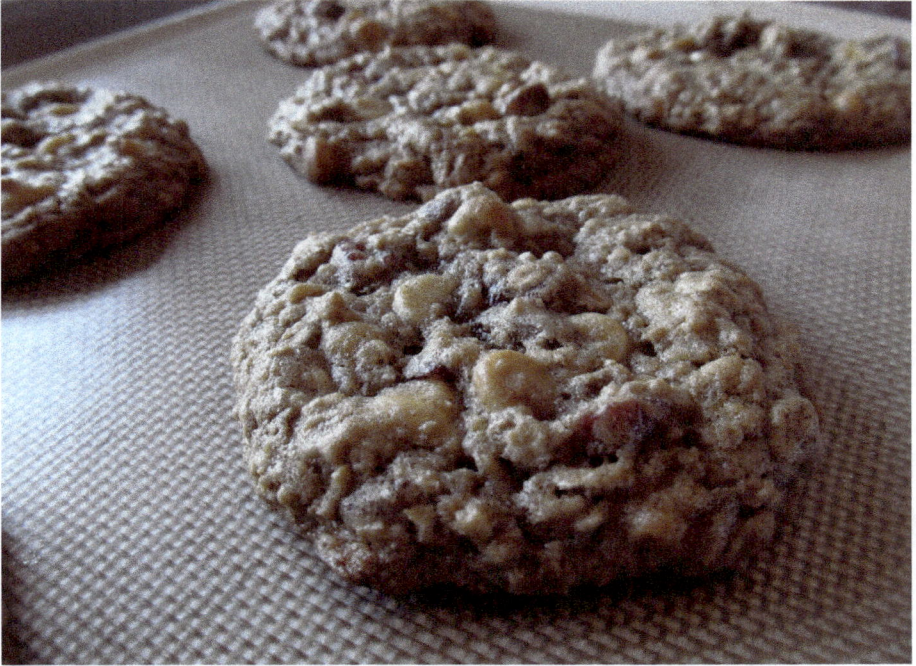

Sides, Salads, and Soups

Rich Chicken and Small Pasta Broth

Prep time: 10 minutes | Cook time: 4 hours | Serves 6

6 boneless, skinless chicken thighs

4 stalks celery, cut into ½-inch pieces

4 carrots, cut into 1-inch pieces

1 medium yellow onion, halved

2 garlic cloves, minced

2 bay leaves

Sea salt and freshly ground black pepper, to taste

6 cups low-sodium chicken stock

½ cup stelline pasta

¼ cup chopped fresh flat-leaf parsley

1. Combine the chicken thighs, celery, carrots, onion, and garlic in the slow cooker. Spread with bay leaves and sprinkle with salt and pepper. Toss to mix well.

2. Pour in the chicken stock. Put the lid on and cook on high for 4 hours or until the internal temperature of chicken reaches at least 165ºF (74ºC).

3. In the last 20 minutes of the cooking, remove the chicken from the slow cooker and transfer to a bowl to cool until ready to reserve.
4. Discard the bay leaves and add the pasta to the slow cooker. Put the lid on and cook for 15 minutes or until al dente.
5. Meanwhile, slice the chicken, then put the chicken and parsley in the slow cooker and cook for 5 minutes or until well combined.
6. Pour the soup in a large bowl and serve immediately.

Per Serving

calories: 285 | fat: 10.8g | protein: 27.4g | carbs: 18.8g | fiber: 2.6g | sodium: 815mg

Roasted Root Vegetable Soup

Prep time: 10 minutes | Cook time: 35 minutes | Serves 6

2 parsnips, peeled and sliced

2 carrots, peeled and sliced

2 sweet potatoes, peeled and sliced

1 teaspoon chopped fresh rosemary

1 teaspoon chopped fresh thyme

1 teaspoon sea salt

½ teaspoon freshly ground black pepper

2 tablespoons extra-virgin olive oil

4 cups low-sodium vegetable soup

½ cup grated Parmesan cheese, for garnish (optional)

1. Preheat the oven to 400ºF (205ºC). Line a baking sheet with aluminum foil.
2. Combine the parsnips, carrots, and sweet potatoes in a large bowl, then sprinkle with rosemary, thyme, salt, and pepper, and drizzle with olive oil. Toss to coat the vegetables well.
3. Arrange the vegetables on the baking sheet, then roast in the preheated oven for 30 minutes

or until lightly browned and soft. Flip the vegetables halfway through the roasting.

4. Pour the roasted vegetables with vegetable broth in a food processor, then pulse until creamy and smooth.

5. Pour the puréed vegetables in a saucepan, then warm over low heat until heated through.

6. Spoon the soup in a large serving bowl, then scatter with Parmesan cheese. Serve immediately.

Per Serving

calories: 192 | fat: 5.7g | protein: 4.8g | carbs: 31.5g | fiber: 5.7g | sodium: 797mg

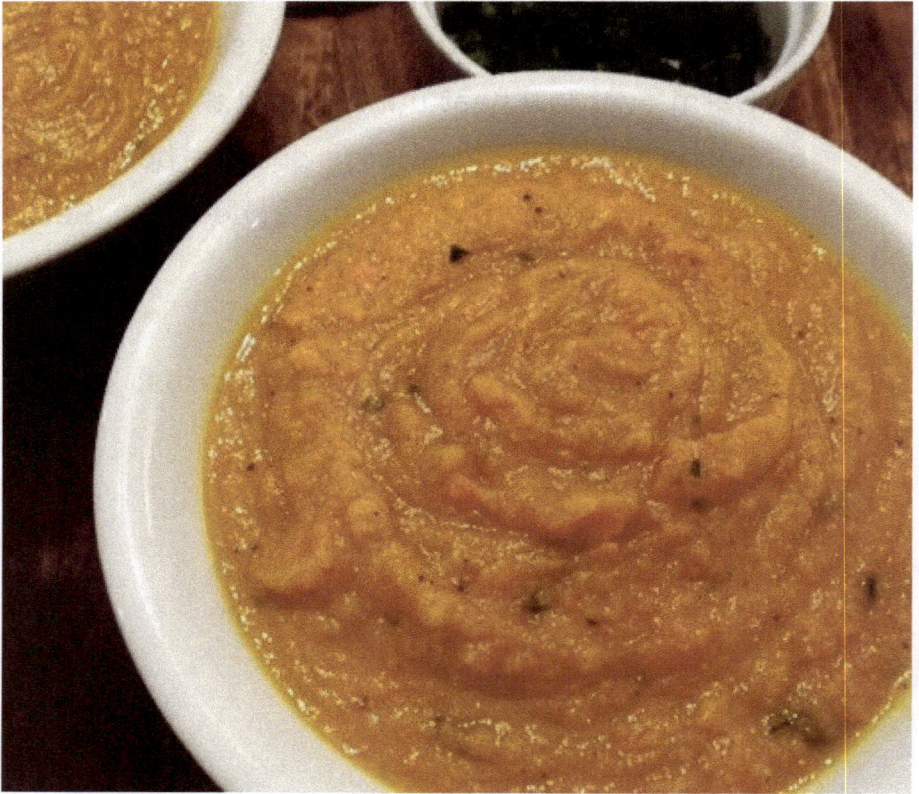

Super Mushroom and Red Wine Soup

Prep time: 40 minutes | Cook time: 35 minutes | Serves 6

2 ounces (57 g) dried morels

2 ounces (57 g) dried porcini

1 tablespoon extra-virgin olive oil

8 ounces (227 g) button mushrooms, chopped

8 ounces (227 g) portobello mushrooms, chopped

3 shallots, finely chopped

2 cloves garlic, minced

1 teaspoon finely chopped fresh thyme

Sea salt and freshly ground pepper, to taste

1⅓ cup dry red wine

4 cups low-sodium chicken broth

½ cup heavy cream

1 small bunch flat-leaf parsley, chopped

1. Put the dried mushrooms in a large bowl and pour in enough water to submerge the mushrooms. Soak for 30 minutes and drain.
2. Heat the olive oil in a stockpot over medium-high heat until shimmering.
3. Add the mushrooms and shallots to the pot and sauté for 10 minutes or until the mushrooms are tender.

4. Add the garlic and sauté for an additional 1 minute or until fragrant. Sprinkle with thyme, salt, and pepper.
5. Pour in the dry red wine and chicken broth. Bring to a boil over high heat.
6. Reduce the heat to low. Simmer for 20 minutes.
7. After simmering, pour half of the soup in a food processor, then pulse until creamy and smooth.
8. Pour the puréed soup back to the pot, then mix in the cream and heat over low heat until heated through.
9. Pour the soup in a large serving bowl and spread with chopped parsley before serving.

Per Serving

calories: 139 | fat: 7.4g | protein: 7.1g | carbs: 14.4g | fiber: 2.8g | sodium: 94mg

Cheesy Roasted Broccolini

Prep time: 5 minutes | Cook time: 10 minutes | Serves 2

1 bunch broccolini (about 5 ounces / 142 g)

1 tablespoon olive oil

½ teaspoon garlic powder

¼ teaspoon salt

2 tablespoons grated Romano cheese

1. Preheat the oven to 400ºF (205ºC). Line a sheet pan with parchment paper.
2. Slice the tough ends off the broccolini and put in a medium bowl. Add the olive oil, garlic powder, and salt and toss to coat well. Arrange the broccolini on the prepared sheet pan.
3. Roast in the preheated oven for 7 minutes, flipping halfway through the cooking time.
4. Remove the pan from the oven and sprinkle the cheese over the broccolini. Using tongs, carefully flip the broccolini over to coat all sides.
5. Return to the oven and cook for an additional 2 to 3 minutes, or until the cheese melts and starts to turn golden. Serve warm.

Per Serving

calories: 114 | fat: 9.0g | protein: 4.0g | carbs: 5.0g | fiber: 2.0g | sodium: 400mg

Orange-Honey Glazed Carrots

Prep time: 10 minutes | Cook time: 15 to 20 minutes | Serves 2

½ pound (227 g) rainbow carrots, peeled

2 tablespoons fresh orange juice

1 tablespoon honey

½ teaspoon coriander

Pinch salt

1. Preheat the oven to 400ºF (205ºC).
2. Cut the carrots lengthwise into slices of even thickness and place in a large bowl.
3. Stir together the orange juice, honey, coriander, and salt in a small bowl. Pour the orange juice mixture over the carrots and toss until well coated.
4. Spread the carrots in a baking dish in a single layer. Roast for 15 to 20 minutes until fork-tender.
5. Let cool for 5 minutes before serving.

Per Serving

calories: 85 | fat: 0g | protein: 1.0g | carbs: 21.0g | fiber: 3.0g | sodium: 156mg

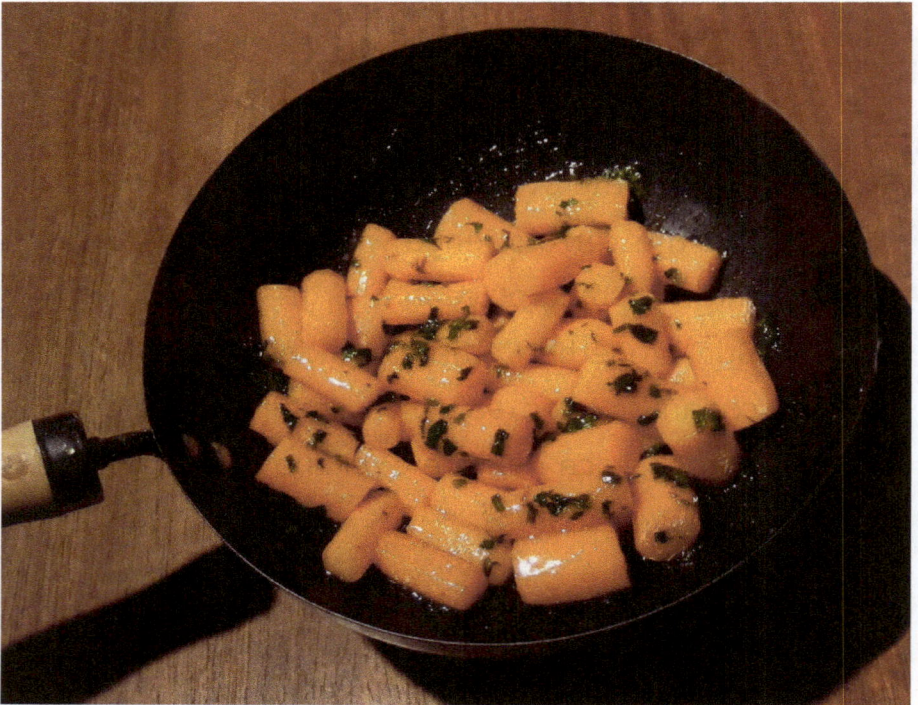

Roasted Cauliflower

Prep time: 10 minutes | Cook time: 20 minutes | Serves 2

½ large head cauliflower, stemmed and broken into florets (about 3 cups)

1 tablespoon olive oil

2 tablespoons freshly squeezed lemon juice

2 tablespoons tahini

1 teaspoon harissa paste Pinch salt

1. Preheat the oven to 400ºF (205ºC). Line a sheet pan with parchment paper.
2. Toss the cauliflower florets with the olive oil in a large bowl and transfer to the sheet pan.
3. Roast in the preheated oven for 15 minutes, flipping the cauliflower once or twice, or until it starts to become golden.
4. Meanwhile, in a separate bowl, combine the lemon juice, tahini, harissa, and salt and stir to mix well.
5. Remove the pan from the oven and toss the cauliflower with the lemon tahini sauce. Return to the oven and roast for another 5 minutes. Serve hot.

Per Serving

calories: 205 | fat: 15.0g | protein: 4.0g | carbs: 15.0g | fiber: 7.0g | sodium: 161mg

Sautéed White Beans with Rosemary

Prep time: 10 minutes | Cook time: 12 minutes | Serves 2

1 tablespoon olive oil

2 garlic cloves, minced

1 (15-ounce / 425-g) can white cannellini beans, drained and rinsed

1 teaspoon minced fresh rosemary plus 1 whole fresh rosemary sprig

¼ teaspoon dried sage

½ cup low-sodium chicken stock

Salt, to taste

1. Heat the olive oil in a saucepan over medium-high heat.
2. Add the garlic and sauté for 30 seconds until fragrant.
3. Add the beans, minced and whole rosemary, sage, and chicken stock and bring the mixture to a boil.
4. Reduce the heat to medium and allow to simmer for 10 minutes, or until most of the liquid is evaporated. If desired, mash some of the beans with a fork to thicken them.

5. Season with salt to taste. Remove the rosemary
    sprig before serving.

Per Serving

calories: 155 | fat: 7.0g | protein: 6.0g | carbs: 17.0g |
fiber: 8.0g | sodium: 153mg

Moroccan Spiced Couscous

Prep time: 10 minutes | Cook time: 8 minutes | Serves 2

1 tablespoon olive oil

¾ cup couscous

¼ teaspoon cinnamon

¼ teaspoon garlic powder

¼ teaspoon salt, plus more as needed

1 cup water

2 tablespoons minced dried apricots

2 tablespoons raisins

2 teaspoons minced fresh parsley

1. Heat the olive oil in a saucepan over medium-high heat until it shimmers.
2. Add the couscous, cinnamon, garlic powder, and salt. Stir for 1 minute to toast the couscous and spices.
3. Add the water, apricots, and raisins and bring the mixture to a boil.
4. Cover and turn off the heat. Allow the couscous to sit for 4 to 5 minutes and then fluff it with a fork. Sprinkle with the fresh parsley. Season with more salt as needed and serve.

Per Serving

calories: 338 | fat: 8.0g | protein: 9.0g | carbs: 59.0g | fiber: 4.0g | sodium: 299mg

Lemon-Tahini Hummus

Prep time: 15 minutes | Cook time: 0 minutes | Serves 6

1 (15-ounce / 425-g) can chickpeas, drained and rinsed

4 tablespoons extra-virgin olive oil, divided

4 to 5 tablespoons tahini (sesame seed paste)

2 lemons, juiced

1 lemon, zested, divided

1 tablespoon minced garlic

Pinch salt

1. In a food processor, combine the chickpeas, 2 tablespoons of olive oil, tahini, lemon juice, half of the lemon zest, and garlic and pulse for up to 1 minute, scraping down the sides of the food processor bowl as necessary.
2. Taste and add salt as needed. Feel free to add 1 teaspoon of water at a time to thin the hummus to a better consistency.
3. Transfer the hummus to a serving bowl. Serve drizzled with the remaining 2 tablespoons of olive oil and remaining half of the lemon zest.

Per Serving

calories: 216 | fat: 15.0g | protein: 5.0g | carbs: 17.0g | fiber: 5.0g | sodium: 12mg

Lemon and Spinach Orzo

Prep time: 5 minutes | Cook time: 10 minutes | Makes 2 cups

1 cup dry orzo

1 (6-ounce / 170-g) bag baby spinach

1 cup halved grape tomatoes

2 tablespoons extra-virgin olive oil

¼ teaspoon salt

Freshly ground black pepper

¾ cup crumbled feta cheese

1 lemon, juiced and zested

1. Bring a medium pot of water to a boil. Stir in the orzo and cook uncovered for 8 minutes. Drain the water, then return the orzo to medium heat.
2. Add the spinach and tomatoes and cook until the spinach is wilted.
3. Sprinkle with the olive oil, salt, and pepper and mix well. Top with the feta cheese, lemon juice and zest, then toss one or two more times and serve.

Per Serving (1 cup)

calories: 610 | fat: 27.0g | protein: 21.0g | carbs: 74.0g | fiber: 6.0g | sodium: 990mg

Zesty Spanish Potato Salad

Prep time: 10 minutes | Cook time: 5 to 7 minutes | Serves 6 to 8

4 russet potatoes, peeled and chopped

3 large hard-boiled eggs, chopped

1 cup frozen mixed vegetables, thawed

½ cup plain, unsweetened, full-fat Greek yogurt

5 tablespoons pitted Spanish olives

½ teaspoon freshly ground black pepper

½ teaspoon dried mustard seed

½ tablespoon freshly squeezed lemon juice

½ teaspoon dried dill Salt, to taste

1. Place the potatoes in a large pot of water and boil for 5 to 7 minutes, until just fork-tender, checking periodically for doneness. You don't have to overcook them.

2. Meanwhile, in a large bowl, mix the eggs, vegetables, yogurt, olives, pepper, mustard, lemon juice, and dill. Season with salt to taste. Once the potatoes are cooled somewhat, add them to the large bowl, then toss well and serve.

Per Serving

calories: 192 | fat: 5.0g | protein: 9.0g | carbs: 30.0g | fiber: 2.0g | sodium: 59mg

Sandwiches, Pizzas, and Wraps

Turkish Eggplant and Tomatoes Pide with Mint

Prep time: 1 day 40 minutes | Cook time: 20 minutes | Makes 6 pides

Dough:

3 cups almond flour

2 teaspoons raw honey

½ teaspoon instant or rapid-rise yeast

1¹⌷ cups ice water

1 tablespoon extra-virgin olive oil

1½ teaspoons sea salt

Eggplant and Tomato Toppings:

28 ounces (794 g) whole tomatoes, peeled and puréed

5 tablespoons extra-virgin olive oil, divided

1 pound (454 g) eggplant, cut into ½-inch pieces

½ red bell pepper, chopped

Sea salt and ground black pepper, to taste

3 garlic cloves, minced

¼ teaspoon red pepper flakes

½ teaspoon smoked paprika

6 tablespoons minced
fresh mint, divided

1½ cups crumbled feta
cheese

Make the Dough

1. Combine the flour, yeast, and honey in a food processor, pulse to combine well. Gently add water while pulsing. Let the dough sit for 10 minutes.
2. Mix the olive oil and salt in the dough and knead the dough until smooth. Wrap in plastic and refrigerate for at least 1 day.

Make the Toppings

3. Heat 2 tablespoons of olive oil in a nonstick skillet over medium-high heat until shimmering.
4. Add the bell pepper, eggplant, and ½ teaspoon of salt. Sauté for 6 minutes or until the eggplant is lightly browned.
5. Add the red pepper flakes, paprika, and garlic. Sauté for 1 minute or until fragrant.

6. Pour in the puréed tomatoes. Bring to a simmer, then cook for 10 minutes or until the mixture is thickened into about 3½ cups.

7. Turn off the heat and mix in 4 tablespoons of mint, salt, and ground black pepper. Set them aside until ready to use.

Make the Turkish Pide

8. Preheat the oven to 500ºF (260ºC). Line three baking sheets with parchment papers.

9. On a clean work surface, divide and shape the dough into six 14 by 5- inch ovals. Transfer the dough to the baking sheets.

10. Brush them with 3 tablespoons of olive oil and spread the eggplant mixture and feta cheese on top.

11. Bake in the preheated oven for 12 minutes or until golden brown. Rotate the pide halfway through the baking time.

12. Remove the pide from the oven and spread with remaining mint and serve immediately.

Per Serving (1 pide)

calories: 500 | fat: 22.1g | protein: 8.0g | carbs: 69.7g | fiber: 5.8g | sodium: 1001mg

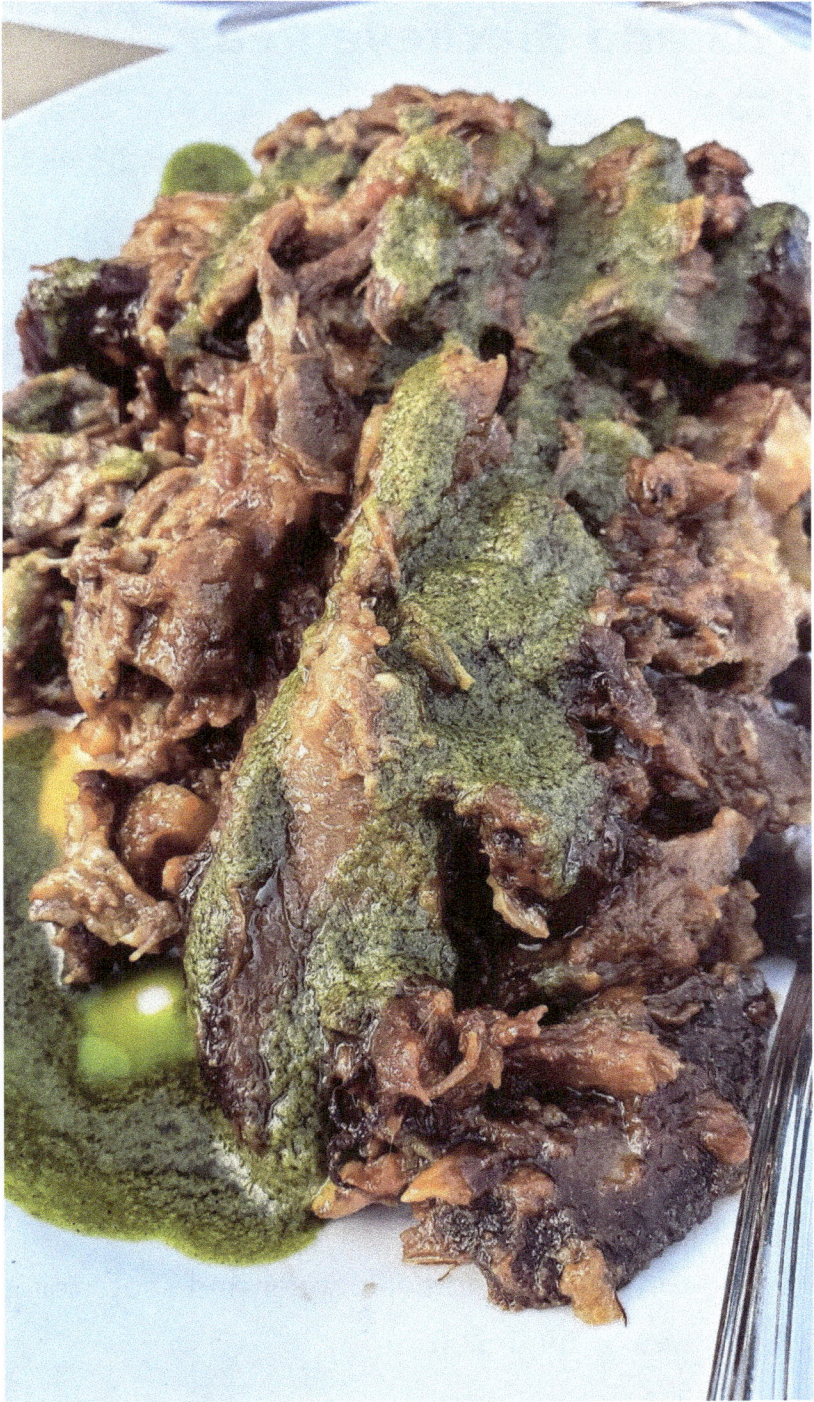

Veg Mix and Blackeye Pea Burritos

Prep time: 15 minutes | Cook time: 40 minutes | Makes 6 burritos

1 teaspoon olive oil

1 red onion, diced

2 garlic cloves, minced

1 zucchini, chopped

1 tomato, diced

1 bell pepper, any color, deseeded and diced

1 (14-ounce / 397-g) can blackeye peas

2 teaspoons chili powder

Sea salt, to taste

6 whole-grain tortillas

1. Preheat the oven to 325ºF (160ºC).
2. Heat the olive oil in a nonstick skillet over medium heat or until shimmering.
3. Add the onion and sauté for 5 minutes or until translucent.
4. Add the garlic and sauté for 30 seconds or until fragrant.
5. Add the zucchini and sauté for 5 minutes or until tender.
6. Add the tomato and bell pepper and sauté for 2 minutes or until soft.

7. Fold in the black peas and sprinkle them with chili powder and salt. Stir to mix well.

8. Place the tortillas on a clean work surface, then top them with sautéed vegetables mix.

9. Fold one ends of tortillas over the vegetable mix, then tuck and roll them into burritos.

10. Arrange the burritos in a baking dish, seam side down, then pour the juice remains in the skillet over the burritos.

11. Bake in the preheated oven for 25 minutes or until golden brown.

12. Serve immediately.

Per Serving

calories: 335 | fat: 16.2g | protein: 12.1g | carbs: 8.3g | fiber: 8.0g | sodium: 214mg

Tuna and Olive Salad Sandwiches

Prep time: 10 minutes | Cook time: 0 minutes | Serves 4

3 tablespoons freshly squeezed lemon juice

2 tablespoons extra-virgin olive oil

1 garlic clove, minced

½ teaspoon freshly ground black pepper

2 (5-ounce / 142-g) cans tuna, drained

1 (2.25-ounce / 64-g) can sliced olives, any green or black variety

½ cup chopped fresh fennel, including fronds

8 slices whole-grain crusty bread

1. In a medium bowl, whisk together the lemon juice, oil, garlic, and pepper. Add the tuna, olives and fennel to the bowl. Using a fork, separate the tuna into chunks and stir to incorporate all the ingredients.

2. Divide the tuna salad equally among 4 slices of bread. Top each with the remaining bread slices.

3. Let the sandwiches sit for at least 5 minutes so the zesty filling can soak into the bread before serving.

Per Serving

calories: 952 | fat: 17.0g | protein: 165.0g | carbs: 37.0g
| fiber: 7.0g | sodium: 2572mg

Open-Faced Margherita Sandwiches

Prep time: 10 minutes | Cook time: 5 minutes | Serves 4

2 (6- to 7-inch) whole-wheat submarine or hoagie rolls, sliced open horizontally

1 tablespoon extra-virgin olive oil

1 garlic clove, halved

1 large ripe tomato, cut into 8 slices

¼ teaspoon dried oregano

1 cup fresh Mozzarella, sliced

¼ cup lightly packed fresh basil leaves, torn into small pieces

¼ teaspoon freshly ground black pepper

1. Preheat the broiler to High with the rack 4 inches under the heating element.
2. Put the sliced bread on a large, rimmed baking sheet and broil for 1 minute, or until the bread is just lightly toasted. Remove from the oven.
3. Brush each piece of the toasted bread with the oil, and rub a garlic half over each piece.
4. Put the toasted bread back on the baking sheet. Evenly divide the tomato slices on each piece.

Sprinkle with the oregano and top with the cheese.

5. Place the baking sheet under the broiler. Set the timer for 1½ minutes, but check after 1 minute. When the cheese is melted and the edges are just starting to get dark brown, remove the sandwiches from the oven.

6. Top each sandwich with the fresh basil and pepper before serving.

Per Serving

calories: 93 | fat: 2.0g | protein: 10.0g | carbs: 8.0g | fiber: 2.0g | sodium: 313mg

Roasted Vegetable Panini

Prep time: 10 minutes | Cook time: 15 minutes | Serves 4

2 tablespoons extra-virgin olive oil, divided

1½ cups diced broccoli

1 cup diced zucchini

¼ cup diced onion

¼ teaspoon dried oregano

⅛ teaspoon kosher or sea salt

⅛ teaspoon freshly ground black pepper

1 (12-ounce / 340-g) jar roasted red peppers, drained and finely chopped

2 tablespoons grated Parmesan or Asiago cheese

1 cup fresh Mozzarella (about 4 ounces / 113 g), sliced

1 (2-foot-long) whole-grain Italian loaf, cut into

4 equal lengths Cooking spray

1. Place a large, rimmed baking sheet in the oven. Preheat the oven to 450ºF (235ºC) with the baking sheet inside.
2. In a large bowl, stir together 1 tablespoon of the oil, broccoli, zucchini, onion, oregano, salt and pepper.

3. Remove the baking sheet from the oven and spritz the baking sheet with cooking spray. Spread the vegetable mixture on the baking sheet and roast for 5 minutes, stirring once halfway through cooking.

4. Remove the baking sheet from the oven. Stir in the red peppers and Parmesan cheese.

5. In a large skillet over medium-high heat, heat the remaining 1 tablespoon of the oil.

6. Cut open each section of bread horizontally, but don't cut all the way through. Fill each with the vegetable mix (about ½ cup), and layer 1 ounce (28 g) of sliced Mozzarella cheese on top. Close the sandwiches, and place two of them on the skillet. Place a heavy object on top and grill for 2½ minutes. Flip the sandwiches and grill for another 2½ minutes.

7. Repeat the grilling process with the remaining two sandwiches.

8. Serve hot.

Per Serving

calories: 116 | fat: 4.0g | protein: 12.0g | carbs: 9.0g | fiber: 3.0g | sodium: 569mg

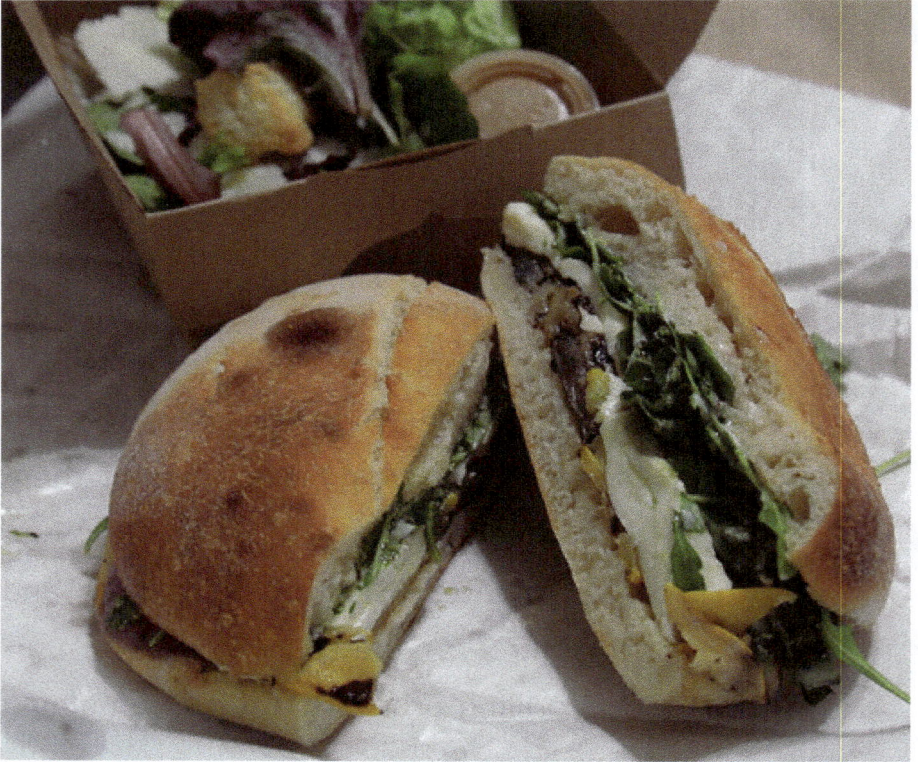

White Pizzas with Arugula and Spinach

Prep time: 10 minutes | Cook time: 20 minutes | Serves 4

1 pound (454 g) refrigerated fresh pizza dough

2 tablespoons extra-virgin olive oil, divided

½ cup thinly sliced onion

2 garlic cloves, minced

3 cups baby spinach

3 cups arugula

1 tablespoon water

¼ teaspoon freshly ground black pepper

1 tablespoon freshly squeezed lemon juice

½ cup shredded Parmesan cheese

½ cup crumbled goat cheese

Cooking spray

1. Preheat the oven to 500ºF (260ºC). Spritz a large, rimmed baking sheet with cooking spray.
2. Take the pizza dough out of the refrigerator.
3. Heat 1 tablespoon of the oil in a large skillet over medium heat. Add the onion to the skillet and cook for 4 minutes, stirring constantly. Add the garlic and cook for 1 minute, stirring constantly.

4. Stir in the spinach, arugula, water and pepper. Cook for about 2 minutes, stirring constantly, or until all the greens are coated with oil and they start to cook down. Remove the skillet from the heat and drizzle with the lemon juice.

5. On a lightly floured work surface, form the pizza dough into a 12-inch circle or a 10-by-12-inch rectangle, using a rolling pin or by stretching with your hands.

6. Place the dough on the prepared baking sheet. Brush the dough with the remaining 1 tablespoon of the oil. Spread the cooked greens on top of the dough to within ½ inch of the edge. Top with the Parmesan cheese and goat cheese.

7. Bake in the preheated oven for 10 to 12 minutes, or until the crust starts to brown around the edges.

8. Remove from the oven and transfer the pizza to a cutting board. Cut into eight pieces before serving.

Per Serving

calories: 521 | fat: 31.0g | protein: 23.0g | carbs: 38.0g | fiber: 4.0g | sodium: 1073mg

Za'atar Pizza

Prep time: 10 minutes | Cook time: 1o to 12 minutes | Serves 4 to 6

1 sheet puff pastry $\frac{1}{3}$ cup za'atar seasoning

¼ cup extra-virgin olive oil

1. Preheat the oven to 350ºF (180ºC). Line a baking sheet with parchment paper.
2. Place the puff pastry on the prepared baking sheet. Cut the pastry into desired slices.
3. Brush the pastry with the olive oil. Sprinkle with the za'atar seasoning.
4. Put the pastry in the oven and bake for 10 to 12 minutes, or until edges are lightly browned and puffed up.
5. Serve warm.

Per Serving

calories: 374 | fat: 30.0g | protein: 3.0g | carbs: 20.0g | fiber: 1.0g | sodium: 166mg

Zucchini Hummus Wraps

Prep time: 15 minutes | Cook time: 6 minutes | Serves 2

1 zucchini, ends removed, thinly sliced lengthwise

½ teaspoon dried oregano

¼ teaspoon freshly ground black pepper

¼ teaspoon garlic powder

¼ cup hummus

2 whole wheat tortillas

2 Roma tomatoes, cut lengthwise into slices

1 cup chopped kale

2 tablespoons chopped red onion

½ teaspoon ground cumin

1. In a skillet over medium heat, add the zucchini slices and cook for 3 minutes per side. Sprinkle with the oregano, pepper, and garlic powder and remove from the heat.

2. Spread 2 tablespoons of hummus on each tortilla. Lay half the zucchini in the center of each tortilla. Top with tomato slices, kale, red onion, and ¼ teaspoon of cumin. Wrap tightly and serve.

Per Serving

calories: 248 | fat: 8.1g | protein: 9.1g | carbs: 37.1g | fiber: 8.1g | sodium: mg

Beans, Grains, and Pastas

Spaghetti with Pine Nuts and Cheese

Prep time: 10 minutes | Cook time: 11 minutes | Serves 4 to 6

8 ounces (227 g) spaghetti

4 tablespoons almond butter

1 teaspoon freshly ground black pepper

½ cup pine nuts

1 cup fresh grated Parmesan cheese, divided

1. Bring a large pot of salted water to a boil. Add the pasta and cook for 8 minutes.
2. In a large saucepan over medium heat, combine the butter, black pepper, and pine nuts. Cook for 2 to 3 minutes, or until the pine nuts are lightly toasted.
3. Reserve ½ cup of the pasta water. Drain the pasta and place it into the pan with the pine nuts.
4. Add ¾ cup of the Parmesan cheese and the reserved pasta water to the pasta and toss everything together to evenly coat the pasta.

5. Transfer the pasta to a serving dish and top with the remaining ¼ cup of the Parmesan cheese. Serve immediately.

Per Serving

calories: 542 | fat: 32.0g | protein: 20.0g | carbs: 46.0g | fiber: 2.0g | sodium: 552mg

Creamy Garlic Parmesan Chicken Pasta

Prep time: 5 minutes | Cook time: 15 minutes | Serves 4

3 tablespoons extra-virgin olive oil

2 boneless, skinless chicken breasts, cut into thin strips

1 large onion, thinly sliced

3 tablespoons garlic, minced

1½ teaspoons salt

1 pound (454 g) fettuccine pasta

1 cup heavy whipping cream

¾ cup freshly grated Parmesan cheese, divided

½ teaspoon freshly ground black pepper

1. In a large skillet over medium heat, heat the olive oil. Add the chicken and cook for 3 minutes.
2. Add the onion, garlic and salt to the skillet. Cook for 7 minutes, stirring occasionally.
3. Meanwhile, bring a large pot of salted water to a boil and add the pasta, then cook for 7 minutes.
4. While the pasta is cooking, add the heavy cream, ½ cup of the Parmesan cheese and

black pepper to the chicken. Simmer for 3 minutes.

5. Reserve ½ cup of the pasta water. Drain the pasta and add it to the chicken cream sauce.

6. Add the reserved pasta water to the pasta and toss together. Simmer for 2 minutes. Top with the remaining ¼ cup of the Parmesan cheese and serve warm.

Per Serving

calories: 879 | fat: 42.0g | protein: 35.0g | carbs: 90.0g | fiber: 5.0g | sodium: 1336mg

Bulgur Pilaf with Garbanzo

Prep time: 5 minutes | Cook time: 20 minutes | Serves 4 to 6

3 tablespoons extra-virgin olive oil

1 large onion, chopped

1 (1-pound / 454-g) can garbanzo beans, rinsed and drained

2 cups bulgur wheat, rinsed and drained

1½ teaspoons salt

½ teaspoon cinnamon

4 cups water

1. In a large pot over medium heat, heat the olive oil. Add the onion and cook for 5 minutes.
2. Add the garbanzo beans and cook for an additional 5 minutes.
3. Stir in the remaining ingredients.
4. Reduce the heat to low. Cover and cook for 10 minutes.
5. When done, fluff the pilaf with a fork. Cover and let sit for another 5 minutes before serving.

Per Serving

calories: 462 | fat: 13.0g | protein: 15.0g | carbs: 76.0g | fiber: 19.0g | sodium: 890mg

Pearl Barley Risotto with Parmesan Cheese

Prep time: 5 minutes | Cook time: 20 minutes | Serves 6

4 cups low-sodium or no-salt-added vegetable broth

1 tablespoon extra-virgin olive oil

1 cup chopped yellow onion

2 cups uncooked pearl barley

½ cup dry white wine

1 cup freshly grated Parmesan cheese, divided

¼ teaspoon kosher or sea salt

¼ teaspoon freshly ground black pepper

Fresh chopped chives and lemon wedges, for serving (optional)

1. Pour the broth into a medium saucepan and bring to a simmer.
2. Heat the olive oil in a large stockpot over medium-high heat. Add the onion and cook for about 4 minutes, stirring occasionally.
3. Add the barley and cook for 2 minutes, stirring, or until the barley is toasted. Pour in the wine and cook for about 1 minute, or until most of the liquid evaporates. Add 1 cup of the warm

broth into the pot and cook, stirring, for about 2 minutes, or until most of the liquid is absorbed.

4. Add the remaining broth, 1 cup at a time, cooking until each cup is absorbed (about 2 minutes each time) before adding the next. The last addition of broth will take a bit longer to absorb, about 4 minutes.

5. Remove the pot from the heat, and stir in ½ cup of the cheese, and the salt and pepper.

6. Serve with the remaining ½ cup of the cheese on the side, along with the chives and lemon wedges (if desired).

Per Serving

calories: 421 | fat: 11.0g | protein: 15.0g | carbs: 67.0g | fiber: 11.0g | sodium: 641mg

Israeli Couscous with Asparagus

Prep time: 5 minutes | Cook time: 25 minutes | Serves 6

1½ pounds (680 g) asparagus spears, ends trimmed and stalks chopped into 1-inch pieces

1 garlic clove, minced

1 tablespoon extra-virgin olive oil

¼ teaspoon freshly ground black pepper

1¾ cups water

1 (8-ounce / 227-g) box uncooked whole-wheat or regular

Israeli couscous

(about 1¼ cups)

¼ teaspoon kosher salt

1 cup garlic-and-herb goat cheese, at room temperature

1. Preheat the oven to 425ºF (220ºC).
2. In a large bowl, stir together the asparagus, garlic, oil, and pepper. Spread the asparagus on a large, rimmed baking sheet and roast for 10 minutes, stirring a few times. Remove the pan from the oven, and spoon the asparagus into a large serving bowl. Set aside.

3. While the asparagus is roasting, bring the water to a boil in a medium saucepan. Add the couscous and season with salt, stirring well.

4. Reduce the heat to medium-low. Cover and cook for 12 minutes, or until the water is absorbed.

5. Pour the hot couscous into the bowl with the asparagus. Add the goat cheese and mix thoroughly until completely melted.

6. Serve immediately.

Per Serving

calories: 103 | fat: 2.0g | protein: 6.0g | carbs: 18.0g | fiber: 5.0g | sodium: 343mg

Freekeh Pilaf with Dates and Pistachios

Prep time: 10 minutes | Cook time: 10 minutes | Serves 4 to 6

2 tablespoons extra-virgin olive oil, plus extra for drizzling

1 shallot, minced

1½ teaspoons grated fresh ginger

¼ teaspoon ground coriander

¼ teaspoon ground cumin

Salt and pepper, to taste

1¾ cups water

1½ cups cracked freekeh, rinsed

3 ounces (85 g) pitted dates, chopped

¼ cup shelled pistachios, toasted and coarsely chopped

1½ tablespoons lemon juice

¼ cup chopped fresh mint

1. Set the Instant Pot to Sauté mode and heat the olive oil until shimmering.
2. Add the shallot, ginger, coriander, cumin, salt, and pepper to the pot and cook for about 2 minutes, or until the shallot is softened. Stir in the water and freekeh.

3. Secure the lid. Select the Manual mode and set the cooking time for 4 minutes at High Pressure. Once cooking is complete, do a quick pressure release. Carefully open the lid.
4. Add the dates, pistachios and lemon juice and gently fluff the freekeh with a fork to combine. Season to taste with salt and pepper.
5. Transfer to a serving dish and sprinkle with the mint. Serve drizzled with extra olive oil.

Per Serving

calories: 280 | fat: 8.0g | protein: 8.0g | carbs: 46.0g | fiber: 9.0g | sodium: 200mg

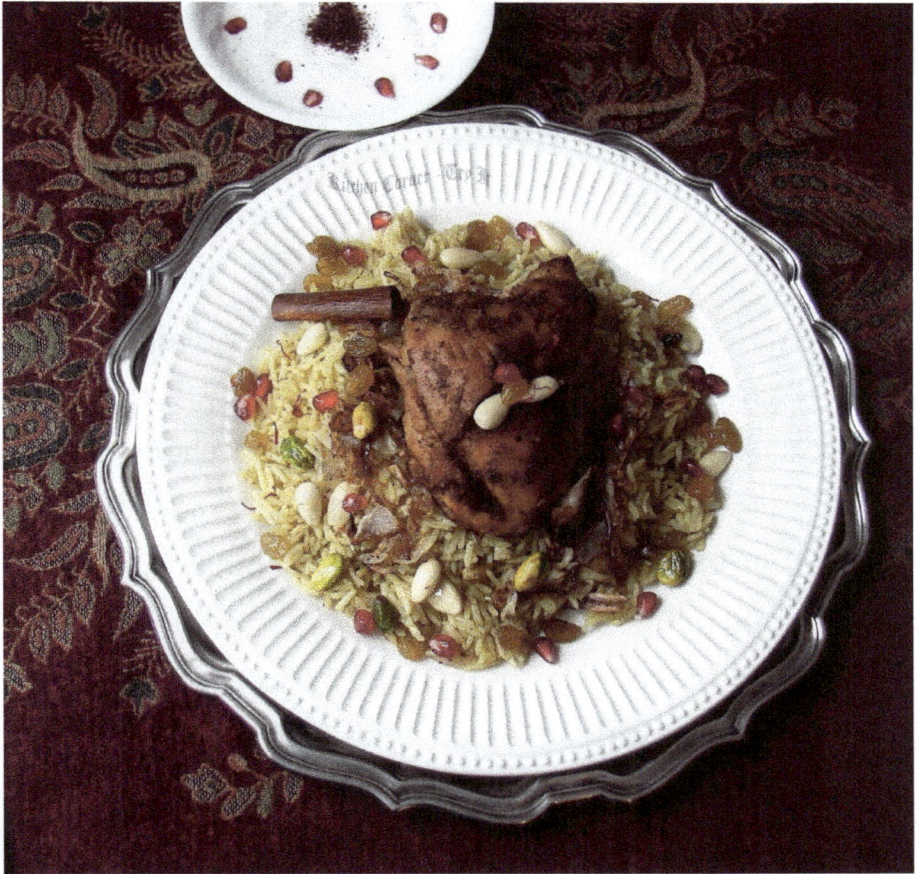

Quinoa with Baby Potatoes and Broccoli

Prep time: 5 minutes | Cook time: 10 minutes | Serves 4

2 tablespoons olive oil	2 cups cooked quinoa
1 cup baby potatoes, cut in half	Zest of 1 lemon
1 cup broccoli florets	Sea salt and freshly ground pepper, to taste

1. Heat the olive oil in a large skillet over medium heat until shimmering.
2. Add the potatoes and cook for about 6 to 7 minutes, or until softened and golden brown. Add the broccoli and cook for about 3 minutes, or until tender.
3. Remove from the heat and add the quinoa and lemon zest. Season with salt and pepper to taste, then serve.

Per Serving

calories: 205 | fat: 8.6g | protein: 5.1g | carbs: 27.3g | fiber: 3.7g | sodium: 158mg

Black-Eyed Pea and Vegetable Stew

Prep time: 15 minutes | Cook time: 40 minutes | Serves 2

½ cup black-eyed peas, soaked in water overnight

3 cups water, plus more as needed

1 large carrot, peeled and cut into ½-inch pieces (about ¾ cup)

1 large beet, peeled and cut into ½-inch pieces (about ¾ cup)

¼ teaspoon turmeric

¼ teaspoon cayenne pepper

¼ teaspoon ground cumin seeds, toasted

¼ cup finely chopped parsley

¼ teaspoon salt (optional)

½ teaspoon fresh lime juice

1. Pour the black-eyed peas and water into a large pot, then cook over medium heat for 25 minutes.
2. Add the carrot and beet to the pot and cook for 10 minutes more, adding more water as needed.

3. Add the turmeric, cayenne pepper, cumin, and parsley to the pot and cook for another 6 minutes, or until the vegetables are softened. Stir the mixture periodically. Season with salt, if desired.

4. Serve drizzled with the fresh lime juice.

Per Serving

calories: 89 | fat: 0.7g | protein: 4.1g | carbs: 16.6g | fiber: 4.5g | sodium: 367mg

Chickpea Salad with Tomatoes and Basil

Prep time: 5 minutes | Cook time: 45 minutes | Serves 2

1 cup dried chickpeas, rinsed

1 quart water, or enough to cover the chickpeas by 3 to 4 inches

1½ cups halved grape tomatoes

1 cup chopped fresh basil leaves

2 to 3 tablespoons balsamic vinegar

½ teaspoon garlic powder

½ teaspoon salt, or more to taste

1. In your Instant Pot, combine the chickpeas and water.

2. Secure the lid. Select the Manual mode and set the cooking time for 45 minutes at High Pressure.

3. Once cooking is complete, do a natural pressure release for 20 minutes, then release any remaining pressure. Carefully open the lid and drain the chickpeas. Refrigerate to cool (unless you want to serve this warm, which is good, too).

4. While the chickpeas cool, in a large bowl, stir together the basil, tomatoes, vinegar, garlic powder, and salt. Add the beans, stir to combine, and serve.

Per Serving

calories: 395 | fat: 6.0g | protein: 19.8g | carbs: 67.1g | fiber: 19.0g | sodium: 612mg

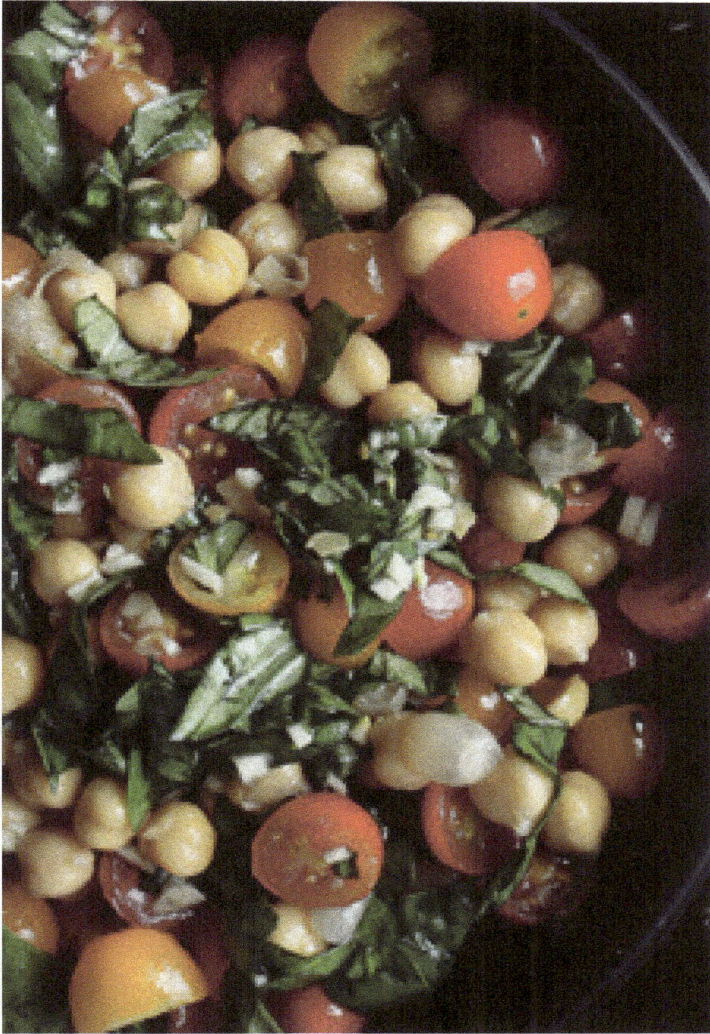

Mediterranean Lentils

Prep time: 7 minutes | Cook time: 24 minutes | Serves 2

1 tablespoon olive oil

1 small sweet or yellow onion, diced

1 garlic clove, diced

1 teaspoon dried oregano

½ teaspoon ground cumin

½ teaspoon dried parsley

½ teaspoon salt, plus more as needed

¼ teaspoon freshly ground black pepper, plus more as needed

1 tomato, diced

1 cup brown or green lentils

2½ cups vegetable stock

1 bay leaf

1. Set your Instant Pot to Sauté and heat the olive oil until it shimmers.
2. Add the onion and cook for 3 to 4 minutes until soft. Turn off the Instant Pot and add the garlic, oregano, cumin, parsley, salt, and pepper. Cook until fragrant, about 1 minute.
3. Stir in the tomato, lentils, stock, and bay leaf.

4. Lock the lid. Select the Manual mode and set the cooking time for 18 minutes at High Pressure.

5. When the timer beeps, perform a natural pressure release for 10 minutes, then release any remaining pressure. Carefully open the lid.

6. Remove and discard the bay leaf. Taste and season with more salt and pepper, as needed. If there's too much liquid remaining, select Sauté and cook until it evaporates.

7. Serve warm.

Per Serving

calories: 426 | fat: 8.1g | protein: 26.2g | carbs: 63.8g | fiber: 31.0g | sodium: 591mg

Mediterranean-Style Beans and Greens

Prep time: 10 minutes | Cook time: 15 minutes | Serves 2

1 (14.5-ounce / 411-g) can diced tomatoes with juice

1 (15-ounce / 425-g) can cannellini beans, drained and rinsed

2 tablespoons chopped green olives, plus 1 or 2 sliced for garnish

¼ cup vegetable broth, plus more as needed

1 teaspoon extra-virgin olive oil

2 cloves garlic, minced

4 cups arugula

¼ cup freshly squeezed lemon juice

1. In a medium saucepan, bring the tomatoes, beans, and chopped olives to a low boil, adding just enough broth to make the ingredients saucy (you may need more than ¼ cup if your canned tomatoes don't have a lot of juice). Reduce heat to low and simmer for about 5 minutes.

2. Meanwhile, in a large skillet, heat the olive oil over medium-high heat. When the oil is hot and starts to shimmer, add garlic and sauté just

until it starts to turn slightly tan, about 30 seconds. Add the arugula and lemon juice, stirring to coat leaves with the olive oil and juice. Cover, reduce the heat to low, and simmer for 3 to 5 minutes.

3. Serve the beans over the greens and garnish with olive slices.

Per Serving

calories: 262 | fat: 5.9g | protein: 13.2g | carbs: 40.4g | fiber: 9.8g | sodium: 897mg

Rich Cauliflower Alfredo

Prep time: 35 minutes | Cook time: 30 minutes | Serves 4

Cauliflower Alfredo Sauce:

1 tablespoon avocado oil

½ yellow onion, diced

2 cups cauliflower florets

2 garlic cloves, minced

1½ teaspoons miso

1 teaspoon Dijon mustard

Pinch of ground nutmeg

½ cup unsweetened almond milk

1½ tablespoons fresh lemon juice

Fettuccine:

1 tablespoon avocado oil

½ yellow onion, diced

1 cup broccoli florets

1 zucchini, halved lengthwise and cut into ¼-inch-thick half-moons

Sea salt and ground black pepper, to taste

½ cup sun-dried tomatoes, drained if packed in oil

8 ounces (227 g) cooked whole-wheat fettuccine

½ cup fresh basil, cut into ribbons

2 tablespoons
nutritional yeast

Sea salt and ground
black pepper, to taste

Make the Sauce

1. Heat the avocado oil in a nonstick skillet over medium-high heat until shimmering.
2. Add half of the onion to the skillet and sauté for 5 minutes or until translucent.
3. Add the cauliflower and garlic to the skillet. Reduce the heat to low and cook for 8 minutes or until the cauliflower is tender.
4. Pour them in a food processor, add the remaining ingredients for the sauce and pulse to combine well. Set aside.

Make the Fettuccine

5. Heat the avocado oil in a nonstick skillet over medium-high heat.
6. Add the remaining half of onion and sauté for 5 minutes or until translucent.
7. Add the broccoli and zucchini. Sprinkle with salt and ground black pepper, then sauté for 5 minutes or until tender.

8. Add the sun-dried tomatoes, reserved sauce, and fettuccine. Sauté for 3 minutes or until well-coated and heated through.

9. Serve the fettuccine on a large plate and spread with basil before serving.

Per Serving

calories: 288 | fat: 15.9g | protein: 10.1g | carbs: 32.5g | fiber: 8.1g | sodium: 185mg

Vegetable Mains

Ratatouille

Prep time: 10 minutes | Cook time: 6 minutes | Serves 4

2 large zucchinis, sliced

2 medium eggplants, sliced

4 medium tomatoes, sliced

2 small red onions, sliced

4 cloves garlic, chopped

2 tablespoons thyme leaves

2 teaspoons sea salt

1 teaspoon black pepper

2 tablespoons balsamic vinegar

4 tablespoons olive oil

2 cups water

1. Line a springform pan with foil and place the chopped garlic in the bottom.
2. Now arrange the vegetable slices, alternately, in circles.
3. Sprinkle the thyme, pepper and salt over the vegetables. Top with oil and vinegar.
4. Pour a cup of water into the instant pot and place the trivet inside.

5. Secure the lid and cook on Manual function for 6 minutes at High Pressure.

6. Release the pressure naturally and remove the lid.

7. Remove the vegetables along with the tin foil.

8. Serve on a platter and enjoy.

Per Serving

calories: 240 | fat: 14.3g | protein: 4.7g | carbs: 27.5g | fiber: 10.8g | sodium: 1181mg

Mushroom and Potato Teriyaki

Prep time: 10 minutes | Cook time: 18 minutes | Serves 4

¾ large yellow or white onion, chopped

1½ medium carrots, diced

1½ ribs celery, chopped

1 medium portabella mushroom, diced

¾ tablespoon garlic, chopped

2 cups water

1 pound (454 g) white potatoes, peeled and diced

¼ cup tomato paste

½ tablespoon sesame oil

2 teaspoons sesame seeds

½ tablespoon paprika

1 teaspoon fresh rosemary

¾ cups peas

¼ cup fresh parsley for garnishing, chopped

1. Add the oil, sesame seeds, and all the vegetables in the instant pot and Sauté for 5 minutes.
2. Stir in the remaining ingredients and secure the lid.
3. Cook on Manual function for 13 minutes at High Pressure.
4. After the beep, natural release the pressure and remove the lid.
5. Garnish with fresh parsley and serve hot.

Per Serving

calories: 160 | fat: 3.0g | protein: 4.7g | carbs: 30.6g |
fiber: 5.5g | sodium: 52mg

Peanut and Coconut Stuffed Eggplants

Prep time: 15 minutes | Cook time: 9 minutes | Serves 4

1 tablespoon coriander seeds

½ teaspoon cumin seeds

½ teaspoon mustard seeds

2 to 3 tablespoons chickpea flour

2 tablespoons chopped peanuts

2 tablespoons coconut shreds

1-inch ginger, chopped

2 cloves garlic, chopped

1 hot green chili, chopped

½ teaspoon ground cardamom

A pinch of cinnamon

¼ to ½ teaspoon cayenne

½ teaspoon turmeric

½ teaspoon raw sugar

½ to ¾ teaspoon salt

1 teaspoon lemon juice

Water as needed

4 baby eggplants

Fresh Cilantro for garnishing

1. Add the coriander, mustard seeds and cumin in the instant pot.
2. Roast on Sauté function for 2 minutes.

83

3. Add the chickpea flour, nuts and coconut shred to the pot, and roast for 2 minutes.

4. Blend this mixture in a blender, then transfer to a medium-sized bowl.

5. Roughly blend the ginger, garlic, raw sugar, chili, and all the spices in a blender.

6. Add the water and lemon juice to make a paste. Combine it with the dry flour mixture.

7. Cut the eggplants from one side and stuff with the spice mixture.

8. Add 1 cup of water to the instant pot and place the stuffed eggplants inside.

9. Sprinkle some salt on top and secure the lid.

10. Cook on Manual for 5 minutes at High Pressure, then quick release the steam.

11. Remove the lid and garnish with fresh cilantro, then serve hot.

Per Serving

calories: 207 | fat: 4.9g | protein: 7.9g | carbs: 39.6g | fiber: 18.3g | sodium: 315mg

Cauliflower with Sweet Potato

Prep time: 15 minutes | Cook time: 8 minutes | Serves 8

1 small onion

4 tomatoes

4 garlic cloves, chopped

2-inch ginger, chopped

2 teaspoons olive oil

1 teaspoon turmeric

2 teaspoons ground cumin Salt, to taste

1 teaspoon paprika

2 medium sweet potatoes, cubed small

2 small cauliflowers, diced

2 tablespoons fresh cilantro for topping, chopped

1. Blend the tomatoes, garlic, ginger and onion in a blender.
2. Add the oil and cumin in the instant pot and Sauté for 1 minute.
3. Stir in the blended mixture and the remaining spices.
4. Add the sweet potatoes and cook for 5 minutes on Sauté
5. Add the cauliflower chunks and secure the lid.
6. Cook on Manual for 2 minutes at High Pressure.

7. Once done, Quick release the pressure and remove the lid.

8. Stir and serve with cilantro on top.

Per Serving

calories: 76 | fat: 1.6g | protein: 2.7g | carbs: 14.4g | fiber: 3.4g | sodium: 55mg

Potato Curry

Prep time: 10 minutes | Cook time: 30 minutes | Serves 2

2 large potatoes, peeled and diced

1 small onion, peeled and diced

8 ounces (227 g) fresh tomatoes

1 tablespoon olive oil

1 cup water

2 tablespoons garlic cloves, grated

½ tablespoon rosemary

½ tablespoon cayenne pepper

1½ tablespoons thyme

Salt and pepper, to taste

1. Pour a cup of water into the instant pot and place the steamer trivet inside.
2. Place the potatoes and half the garlic over the trivet and sprinkle some salt and pepper on top.
3. Secure the lid and cook on Steam function for 20 minutes.
4. After the beep, natural release the pressure and remove the lid.
5. Put the potatoes to one side and empty the pot.
6. Add the remaining ingredients to the cooker and Sauté for 10 minutes.

7. Use an immerse blender to purée the cooked mixture.

8. Stir in the steamed potatoes and serve hot.

Per Serving

calories: 398 | fat: 7.6g | protein: 9.6g | carbs: 76.2g | fiber: 10.9g | sodium: 111mg

Mushroom, Potato, and Green Bean Mix

Prep time: 10 minutes | Cook time: 18 minutes | Serves 3

1 tablespoon olive oil

½ carrot, peeled and minced

½ celery stalk, minced

½ small onion, minced

1 garlic clove, minced

½ teaspoon dried sage, crushed

½ teaspoon dried rosemary, crushed

4 ounces (113 g) fresh Portabella mushrooms, sliced

4 ounces (113 g) fresh white mushrooms, sliced

¼ cup red wine

¾ cup fresh green beans, trimmed and chopped

1 cup tomatoes, chopped

½ cup tomato paste

½ tablespoon balsamic vinegar

3 cups water

Salt and freshly ground black pepper to taste

2 ounces (57 g) frozen peas

½ lemon juice

2 tablespoons fresh cilantro for garnishing, chopped

1 Yukon Gold potato, peeled
and diced

1. Put the oil, onion, tomatoes and celery into the instant pot and Sauté for 5 minutes.
2. Stir in the herbs and garlic and cook for 1 minute.
3. Add the mushrooms and sauté for 5 minutes. Stir in the wine and cook for a further 2 minutes
4. Add the diced potatoes and mix. Cover the pot with a lid and let the potatoes cook for 2-3 minutes.
5. Now add the green beans, carrots, tomato paste, peas, salt, pepper, water and vinegar.
6. Secure the lid and cook on Manual function for 8 minutes at High Pressure with the pressure valve in the sealing position.
7. Do a Quick release and open the pot, stir the veggies and then add lemon juice and cilantro, then serve with rice or any other of your choice.

Per Serving

calories: 238 | fat: 5.4g | protein: 8.3g | carbs: 42.7g | fiber: 8.5g | sodium: 113mg

Mushroom Tacos

Prep time: 10 minutes | Cook time: 13 minutes | Serves 3

4 large guajillo chilies

2 teaspoons oil

2 bay leaves

2 large onions, sliced

2 garlic cloves

2 chipotle chillies in adobo sauce

2 teaspoons ground cumin

1 teaspoon dried oregano

1 teaspoon smoked hot paprika

½ teaspoon ground cinnamon, Salt, to taste

¾ cup vegetable broth

1 teaspoon apple cider vinegar

3 teaspoons lime juice

¼ teaspoon sugar

8 ounces (227 g) mushrooms chopped

Whole-wheat tacos, for serving

1. Put the oil, onion, garlic, salt and bay leaves into the instant pot and Sauté for 5 minutes.
2. Blend the half of this mixture, in a blender, with all the spices and chillies.

3. Add the mushrooms to the remaining onions and Sauté for 3 minutes.
4. Pour the blended mixture into the pot and secure the lid.
5. Cook on Manual function for 5 minutes at High Pressure.
6. Once done, Quick release the pressure and remove the lid.
7. Stir well and serve with tacos.

Per Serving

calories: 138 | fat: 4.1g | protein: 5.7g | carbs: 23.8g | fiber: 4.8g | sodium: 208mg

Lentils and Eggplant Curry

Prep time: 10 minutes | Cook time: 22 minutes | Serves 4

¾ cup lentils, soaked and rinsed

1 teaspoon olive oil

½ onion, chopped

4 garlic cloves, chopped

1 teaspoon ginger, chopped

1 hot green chili, chopped

¼ teaspoon turmeric

½ teaspoon ground cumin

2 tomatoes, chopped

1 cup eggplant, chopped

1 cup sweet potatoes, cubed

¾ teaspoon salt

2 cups water

1 cup baby spinach leaves

Cayenne and lemon/lime to taste

Pepper flakes (garnish)

1. Add the oil, garlic, ginger, chili and salt into the instant pot and Sauté for 3 minutes.
2. Stir in the tomatoes and all the spices. Cook for 5 minutes.
3. Add all the remaining ingredients, except the spinach leaves and garnish.
4. Secure the lid and cook on Manual function for 12 minutes at High Pressure.

5. After the beep, release the pressure naturally and remove the lid.

6. Stir in the spinach leaves and let the pot simmer for 2 minutes on Sauté.

7. Garnish with the pepper flakes and serve warm.

Per Serving

calories: 88 | fat: 1.5g | protein: 3.4g | carbs: 17.4g | fiber: 3.3g | sodium: 470mg

Sweet Potato and Tomato Curry

Prep time: 5 minutes | Cook time: 8 minutes | Serves 8

2 large brown onions, finely diced

4 tablespoons olive oil

4 teaspoons salt

4 large garlic cloves, diced

1 red chili, sliced

4 tablespoons cilantro, chopped

4 teaspoons ground cumin

2 teaspoons ground coriander

2 teaspoons paprika

2 pounds (907 g) sweet potato, diced

4 cups chopped, tinned tomatoes

2 cups water

2 cups vegetable stock

Lemon juice and cilantro (garnish)

1. Put the oil and onions into the instant pot and Sauté for 5 minutes.
2. Stir in the remaining ingredients and secure the lid.
3. Cook on Manual function for 3 minutes at High Pressure.
4. Once done, Quick release the pressure and remove the lid.
5. Garnish with cilantro and lemon juice.

6. Serve.

Per Serving

calories: 224 | fat: 8.0g | protein: 4.6g | carbs: 35.9g | fiber: 7.5g | sodium: 1385mg

Veggie Chili

Prep time: 15 minutes | Cook time: 10 minutes | Serves 3

½ tablespoon olive oil

1 small yellow onion, chopped

4 garlic cloves, minced

¾ (15-ounce / 425-g) can diced tomatoes

1 ounce (28 g) sugar-free tomato paste

½ (4-ounce / 113-g) can green chilies with liquid

1 tablespoon Worcestershire sauce

2 tablespoons red chili powder

½ cup carrots, diced

½ cup scallions, chopped

½ cup green bell pepper, chopped

¼ cup peas

1 tablespoon ground cumin

½ tablespoon dried oregano, crushed

Salt and freshly ground black pepper to taste

1. Add the oil, onion, and garlic into the instant pot and Sauté for 5 minutes.
2. Stir in the remaining vegetables and stir-fry for 3 minutes.
3. Add the remaining ingredients and secure the lid.

4. Cook on Manual function for 2 minutes at High Pressure.

5. After the beep, natural release the pressure and remove the lid.

6. Stir well and serve warm.

Per Serving

calories: 106 | fat: 3.9g | protein: 3.4g | carbs: 18.0g | fiber: 6.2g | sodium: 492mg

Fish and Seafood

Dill Baked Sea Bass

Prep time: 10 minutes | Cook time: 10 to 15 minutes | Serves 6

¼ cup olive oil

2 pounds (907 g) sea bass

Sea salt and freshly ground pepper, to taste

1 garlic clove, minced

¼ cup dry white wine

3 teaspoons fresh dill

2 teaspoons fresh thyme

1. Preheat the oven to 425ºF (220ºC).

2. Brush the bottom of a roasting pan with the olive oil. Place the fish in the pan and brush the fish with oil.

3. Season the fish with sea salt and freshly ground pepper. Combine the remaining ingredients and pour over the fish.

4. Bake in the preheated oven for 10 to 15 minutes, depending on the size of the fish.

5. Serve hot.

Per Serving

calories: 224 | fat: 12.1g | protein: 28.1g | carbs: 0.9g | fiber: 0.3g | sodium: 104mg

Breaded Shrimp

Prep time: 10 minutes | Cook time: 4 to 6 minutes | Serves 4

2 large eggs

1 tablespoon water

2 cups seasoned Italian bread crumbs

1 teaspoon salt

1 cup flour

1 pound (454 g) large shrimp (21 to 25), peeled and deveined

Extra-virgin olive oil, as needed

1. In a small bowl, beat the eggs with the water, then transfer to a shallow dish.
2. Add the bread crumbs and salt to a separate shallow dish, then mix well.
3. Place the flour into a third shallow dish.
4. Coat the shrimp in the flour, then the beaten egg, and finally the bread crumbs. Place on a plate and repeat with all of the shrimp.
5. Heat a skillet over high heat. Pour in enough olive oil to coat the bottom of the skillet. Cook the shrimp in the hot skillet for 2 to 3 minutes on each side. Remove and drain on a paper towel. Serve warm.

Per Serving

calories: 714 | fat: 34.0g | protein: 37.0g | carbs: 63.0g | fiber: 3.0g | sodium: 1727mg

Pesto Shrimp over Zoodles

Prep time: 15 minutes | Cook time: 10 minutes | Serves 4

1 pound (454 g) fresh shrimp, peeled and deveined

Salt and freshly ground black pepper, to taste

2 tablespoons extra-virgin olive oil

½ small onion, slivered

8 ounces (227 g) store-bought jarred pesto

¾ cup crumbled goat or feta cheese, plus additional for serving

2 large zucchini, spiralized, for serving

¼ cup chopped flat-leaf Italian parsley, for garnish

1. In a bowl, season the shrimp with salt and pepper. Set aside.
2. In a large skillet, heat the olive oil over medium-high heat. Sauté the onion until just golden, 5 to 6 minutes.
3. Reduce the heat to low and add the pesto and cheese, whisking to combine and melt the cheese. Bring to a low simmer and add the shrimp. Reduce the heat back to low and cover. Cook until the shrimp is cooked through and pink, about 3 to 4 minutes.

4. Serve the shrimp warm over zoodles, garnishing with chopped parsley and additional crumbled cheese.

Per Serving

calories: 491 | fat: 35.0g | protein: 29.0g | carbs: 15.0g | fiber: 4.0g | sodium: 870mg

Salt and Pepper Calamari and Scallops

Prep time: 5 minutes | Cook time: 10 minutes | Serves 4

8 ounces (227 g) calamari steaks, cut into ½-inch-thick rings

8 ounces (227 g) sea scallops

1½ teaspoons salt, divided

1 teaspoon garlic powder

1 teaspoon freshly ground black pepper

1⬚ cup extra-virgin olive oil

2 tablespoons almond butter

1. Place the calamari and scallops on several layers of paper towels and pat dry. Sprinkle with 1 teaspoon of salt and allow to sit for 15 minutes at room temperature. Pat dry with additional paper towels. Sprinkle with pepper and garlic powder.

2. In a deep medium skillet, heat the olive oil and butter over medium-high heat. When the oil is hot but not smoking, add the scallops and calamari in a single layer to the skillet and sprinkle with the remaining ½ teaspoon of salt. Cook for 2 to 4 minutes on each side,

depending on the size of the scallops, until just golden but still slightly opaque in center.

3. Using a slotted spoon, remove from the skillet and transfer to a serving platter. Allow the cooking oil to cool slightly and drizzle over the seafood before serving.

Per Serving

calories: 309 | fat: 25.0g | protein: 18.0g | carbs: 3.0g | fiber: 0g | sodium: 928mg

Baked Cod with Vegetables

Prep time: 15 minutes | Cook time: 25 minutes | Serves 2

1 pound (454 g) thick cod fillet, cut into 4 even portions

¼ teaspoon onion powder (optional)

¼ teaspoon paprika

3 tablespoons extra-virgin olive oil

4 medium scallions

½ cup fresh chopped basil, divided

3 tablespoons minced garlic (optional)

2 teaspoons salt

2 teaspoons freshly ground black pepper

¼ teaspoon dry marjoram (optional)

6 sun-dried tomato slices

½ cup dry white wine

½ cup crumbled feta cheese

1 (15-ounce / 425-g) can oil-packed artichoke hearts, drained

1 lemon, sliced

1 cup pitted kalamata olives

1 teaspoon capers (optional)

4 small red potatoes, quartered

1. Preheat the oven to 375ºF (190ºC).
2. Season the fish with paprika and onion powder (if desired).

3. Heat an ovenproof skillet over medium heat and sear the top side of the cod for about 1 minute until golden. Set aside.

4. Heat the olive oil in the same skillet over medium heat. Add the scallions, ¼ cup of basil, garlic (if desired), salt, pepper, marjoram (if desired), tomato slices, and white wine and stir to combine. Bring to a boil and remove from heat.

5. Evenly spread the sauce on the bottom of skillet. Place the cod on top of the tomato basil sauce and scatter with feta cheese. Place the artichokes in the skillet and top with the lemon slices.

6. Scatter with the olives, capers (if desired), and the remaining ¼ cup of basil. Remove from the heat and transfer to the preheated oven. Bake for 15 to 20 minutes, or until it flakes easily with a fork.

7. Meanwhile, place the quartered potatoes on a baking sheet or wrapped in aluminum foil. Bake in the oven for 15 minutes until fork-tender.

8. Cool for 5 minutes before serving.

Per Serving

calories: 1168 | fat: 60.0g | protein: 63.8g | carbs: 94.0g | fiber: 13.0g | sodium: 4620mg

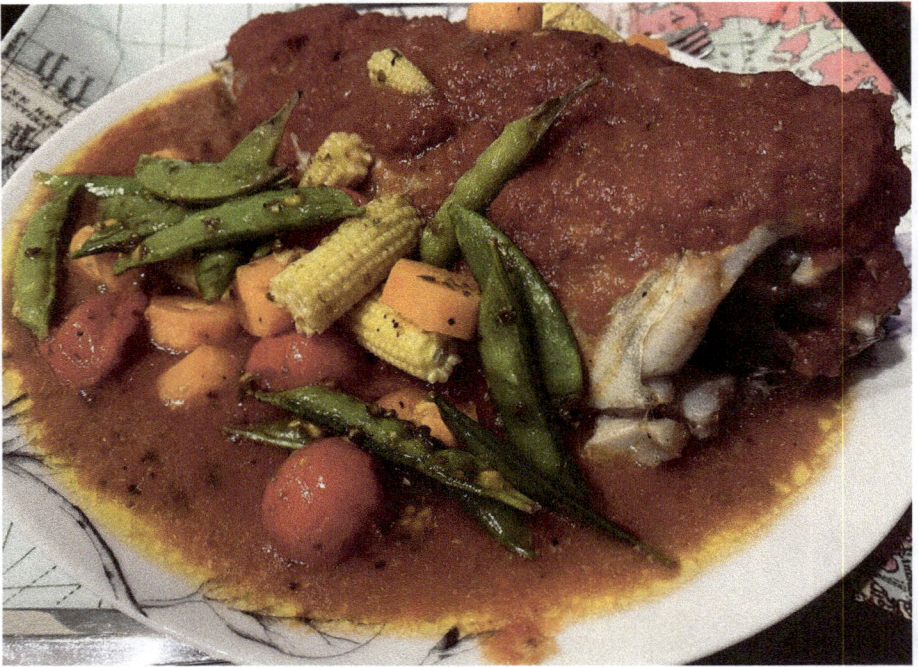